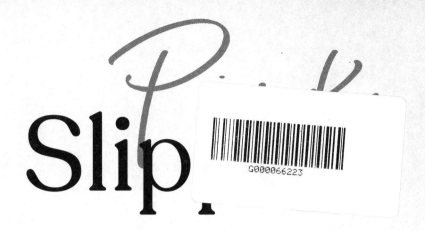

Slip

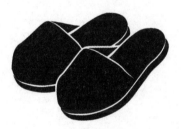

JANE HARDY

Pink Slippers

Mum, dementia and me
A story of hope

Jane Hardy

First published by
Practical Inspiration Publishing, 2019

ISBN 978-1-78860-088-0

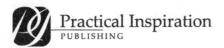

Practical Inspiration
PUBLISHING

Are you caring for a loved one with dementia and don't know where to begin?

This book is dedicated to *you*.

This is what the professionals will fail to tell you.

These are the answers you have been searching for.

No matter how dark your days get, there is always light not too far away.

CONTENTS

INTRODUCTION

This book is about my Mum and me. It's about the experiences we've shared over the past four years, the lessons I've learnt and things I wish I'd known before we started this journey together – hindsight is a wonderful thing.

My Mum, Beth, was diagnosed with vascular dementia and Alzheimer's disease with an MMSE (Mini-Mental State Exam) score of 16 (moderate/severe dementia) at the age of 90. At the time it felt like a death sentence, and I could see no reason for hope. But almost four years later, Mum has a score of 20+, is enjoying life, and her memory and sense of humour are returning and the most important thing of all is that she is content and well cared for.

Even her GP cannot believe her improvement. She is stronger and healthier today and has a far more positive outlook on life. She can read and write again and enjoys speaking to her friends and going out and about.

If you are looking after a loved one with dementia, I hope you'll find the experiences and strategies I've used helpful, and that at least you won't make the same mistakes that I did.

As I tell our story, you'll find helpful ideas and tips along the way, including: how to assist your loved one when they are in hospital; how to choose a suitable care home or carer; how to recognise some of the early signs of dementia; useful gadgets for the home; and general observations and things I've learnt. This journey is not for the faint-hearted. But I truly believe that you can have the same success that I've had with Mum.

One of the best tips I can give you at the outset is *don't* always listen to others. Don't necessarily believe what others tell you. You will be told a lot of things, particularly things that can't be done! I chose to focus on what Mum and I could do together, rather than on what the doctors said couldn't be done. Small steps have led to huge strides.

Pink Slippers is not a scientific 'cure', although I know that Mum is so much better and enjoying a happy and fulfilled life again.

Credentials and experience

To be honest, I don't really have any credentials for writing this book. All I have is four years' experience of looking after Mum, either at her home or mine. I have learnt all I know through mistakes and this book will hopefully ensure that you don't make the same mistakes and discoveries that I did.

I don't have any sponsorship or affinity with any of the products I mention in this book; I'm just sharing with you what I use and what has helped us both.

To be honest...

If I had known the obstacles and challenges we were going to face together, I'm not sure I would have made the same decisions. I adore my Mum and love her with all my heart. I'm so pleased with what we've achieved together. Today, I wouldn't have it any other way, but we have gone through some huge challenges together to get to where we are now.

This book isn't just about Mum; it's about how my life has changed too and if you are caring for a loved one, then your life will also change.

When I took Mum for one of her routine GP appointments, something happened. Mum liked to look good for her doctor's appointment so after several changes of clothing, heaving the wheelchair into the car, getting Mum into the car and strapped in, we finally arrived at the surgery with a minute to spare – phew! We'd made it. The doctor commented on how well Mum looked and then he turned, looked down at my feet and said, 'But I'm rather concerned about your daughter.' Feeling exposed, I looked down and noticed I'd forgotten to change my shoes. I still had my pink slippers on!!

I was *so* obsessed about getting Mum ready, that I hadn't even thought of myself – but *you* need to!

Pink Slippers is for *you*. If you have a friend or relative who has been diagnosed with dementia or whom you suspect has early onset dementia, you're going to need all the help and support you can find. If you're looking for ways to help support yourself and them, then please read on.

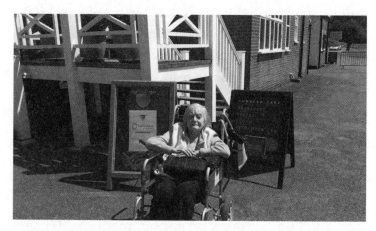

Mum in June 2015.

CHAPTER 1

YOU ARE *NOT* ALONE

Congratulations, you have taken the first step to finding the practical help you need. Remember that you are *not* alone. If you believe you are alone, you are mistaken! I do know what you are going through as I'm living it myself.

This book is for *you*. I appreciate how much you love and care for your friend or relative – you are *fabulous* and please don't forget it. This is my gift to you. Well done for taking on the challenge of looking after a loved one with dementia.

A friend of mine said to me recently, 'My home has become a care home.' She is not wrong and that's part and parcel of your life. You either get on with it, accept it and deal with it, or you get off the merry-go-round *now*.

The journey you face is definitely not a sprint and there is *no* magic wand! Don't rush things, but slowly and surely things really can improve.

Life does *not* prepare you for taking on a loved one with dementia or Alzheimer's disease, or indeed both! However, life does not prepare a loved one to live with this disease either. Unfortunately, dementia is *not* flu, a cold, measles or any other disease; it's a broken brain.

Where there is darkness, there is also light. There is *hope*. As my fabulous friend Jan said to me, 'It's not forever.' Sadly, her Mum Kit died in April 2018. 'Forever' can seem like an awful long time, especially when you are living through it 24/7, but it's never long enough either!

When life throws you a curve ball

What was your life like before you cared for a loved one? Can you remember the old *you*? Was there a time in your life when you didn't have to care for someone and put them first?

Do you now find yourself constantly clock-watching, racing around in constant flight-or-fight mode, waiting for the next problem to arise? Are there appointments to be made and a 'To Do' list so long that you don't know where to begin? Does this sound familiar? Can you relate to this?

How do you feel when you hear the word you dread for the hundredth time and it's still the morning? – (Your name!) Do you get summoned for one thing or another? And when you don't respond immediately, there's hell to pay! Are you ever greeted by someone that has a face like thunder?

My world has become one and the same with Mum. When did that happen? I guess it doesn't really matter when, but I've come to realise that I also matter and need a life too.

Choices we make

Life is about the choices we make. Perhaps you chose to have children, or like me not to have them. Maybe I was too selfish early on in my life. When the time came, my then husband didn't want any children. Maybe I should've said something about wanting children prior to getting married? But, hey, none of that matters now.

So here I am at 57, with no children, divorced, living with my partner and 93-year-old Mum and my two cats, Biscuit and Fudge.

If you were fortunate enough to have children, you knew (I hope) what to expect, right? Well, maybe! You hoped to hold a gorgeous baby in your arms and all their needs would be met by you – from feeding, washing and toileting to all that's involved in bringing up children.

You loved them and watched them grow from the baby stage through the terrible twos and then through their teenage years until eventually they flew the nest and started a life of their own.

When the time came for them to leave home, I'm sure you were upset at first, but you were proud. Your job was complete. Your children had their independence and were living a life of freedom and choice.

There was a point in my life where I could do what I wanted, when I wanted, within reason. Then things changed. Over time, everything has become a blur and I feel like I have 'lost' my identity.

'Doing enough is *never* enough!', so I thought. I have since changed that belief. I now believe anyone can help a dementia patient to improve, have a far better quality of life *and* slow down this horrible disease.

The last four years have been challenging, and this is an understatement. I wish I knew then what I know now, but through the lessons I've learnt, I hope I've become a better person; I know that Mum is a happier and healthier person. But at what cost to me?

Today, whilst writing in the lounge, Mum is just a few feet away from me watching TV – Venus Williams is playing Jelena Ostapenko at Wimbledon. I smile as she is watching avidly, just like she used to. We have come such a long way. The last three years Mum was so disinterested in Wimbledon, which she used to love; in fact, she was disinterested in everything, including life. At one point I thought she was slipping away.

How I've managed to write *Pink Slippers*, have a full-time job and keep sane is something short of a miracle, especially as Mum cannot be left alone for even 10 minutes – hence why I'm writing this book in the lounge with the TV sound blaring as she is somewhat deaf, even with her hearing aids in.

CHAPTER 2

MUM – HISTORY IN THE MAKING

Mum was highly intelligent. She could've done many things with her life. Instead, she and Dad (Peter) decided that her career was to bring up me and my sister. My parents sacrificed a lot. Sarah and I were loved and nurtured; my parents' dreams had come true as we were all so very happy.

Independence was the one thing that Mum wanted for her girls. She gave us the tools and strategies, taught us to dream and 'set us free' to 'spread our wings' and experience this wonderful world. She would *so* hate to think that I had given up anything to support her. But that was my decision, not Mum's.

Mum worked in the library at *The Yorkshire Post* and latterly as a doctor's secretary until the age of 80. She had a full life, loads of friends who she drove around and helped with their shopping etc. She lived alone, from the age of 60.

Mum moved from the 'family' home to her flat when she was 77. I went flat hunting with her and we visited a few. When she walked into what was to become her home, she said out loud, 'This is where I definitely want to live.' Mum was a very determined woman. Once she made up her mind, that was it, no going back. That day was an easy sell for the estate agent!

Mum has always been open and honest and would speak her mind if necessary. Yorkshire born and bred – stubborn is the word I would use!

When she retired at age 80, she worked a couple of days a week at the Windsor Hospice Shop in Sunninghill, Berkshire. She loved working there as she got to make even more friends. Mum never sat still. There was one exception – every year for two weeks in July when Wimbledon was on. Not even wild horses would move her! She was always fiercely independent.

In April 2015, Mum turned 90. She was still driving, socialising, going on outings with her 'club' (a ladies' group of fabulous women), shopping, cooking, reading and cleaning for herself (with the help of the lovely Alison who cleaned once a week). Mum was brilliant at completing the hard *Telegraph* crossword in under 10 minutes. She kept her mind and body active, and loved doing yoga and Pilates. She attended classes once a week, and this was to be a godsend for her later on.

Back in the good old days, I would visit Mum or meet her for a coffee somewhere, or she would visit me once or twice a week. We would chat with each other every night on the phone at 6pm. It was the routine we got into and I was happy. Mum lived her life and I lived mine. Knowing that she was safe and well was always paramount to me.

Mum was as fit as a fiddle. The only medication she was taking was thyroxine, for an over-active thyroid, which she's taken for over 40 years. She does have macular degeneration but taking VitaEyes (twice a day) certainly seemed to have slowed down its progression and she was feeling well.

Mum had cataract operations in both eyes, which were hugely successful. Her consultant ophthalmic, cataract and vitreoretinal surgeon was Mr Vaughan Tanner. It has to be said that Mum never worried about seeing him or having surgery. She found him to be a true professional, yet extremely friendly. She always enjoyed seeing him and thought he was 'pretty dishy too'! Her words, not mine. Mum has a great sense of humour.

Mum was – and still *is* – amazing.

When Mum turned 90, the only thing I insisted on was that she wore an alarm around her neck. It was peace of mind for me; if she had a problem, she could press the button and the Careline Call Centre would call me and I could take action.

It's a bit like having insurance; you hope you never have to use it, but it's good to know it's there. We did have some disagreements about it and 'interesting' conversations but eventually Mum agreed to wear it – but only because I said it was for *my* peace of mind! I always found that if I said to Mum that 'it would make me happy', she would always eventually agree. However, she is somewhat canny and will use this statement on me when it suits her!

CHAPTER 3

THE START OF THE DEMENTIA

At age 89 Mum started to forget a few things, but hey, so do I (at times, living with Mum for the past four or so years I've wondered whether I have early onset dementia, but I don't think the menopause has helped!).

In January 2015, Mum was diagnosed with polymyalgia and came to live with me for two and a half months. She was on steroids and in a lot of pain. It was an awful time and we were back and forth to various consultants and doctors, but slowly she recovered fully. By March 2015 the polymyalgia had calmed down. Mum was good to go home. With the help of daily carers and Meals on Wheels, Mum managed well and I did all her shopping for her, plus a few other bits and pieces, including doctors' appointments.

But in April 2015 after a couple of small falls, Mum had a bad fall in her kitchen – thank goodness for her alarm around her neck. Imagine if she didn't have her alarm on – she would've been on the floor all night, alone, in pain and cold.

According to the staff at the alarm service, when they rang me at 9pm on a Sunday night, they told me that she just kept pressing the button again and again. She was in such a panic.

I immediately called her neighbours, the lovely Vivienne and Ramsey. They went next door immediately and let themselves in using the key safe. Fortunately, I had just fitted a key safe outside Mum's front door. What a stroke of luck that was! (For more information on key safes and alarms for the elderly, please see Chapter 8.)

I drove straight round to Mum's in record time and arrived as the ambulance turned up! Mum was taken to Frimley Park Hospital A&E. We stayed all night until 6am, and the following morning when Mum was taken down to theatre she had a screw inserted into her hip.

Prior to Mum being taken down for surgery, one of the doctors took me to one side and asked me about DNR (Do Not Resuscitate). I hadn't even thought about this, but the doctor was very gentle with me and explained that at Mum's age, something like a heart attack could happen on the operating theatre table. If this happens to you, please do not panic, but take a deep breath and listen to the doctor. Take your time in asking questions, and if you don't understand some or all of the answers, then ask them to explain again; they will be so understanding and caring.

My advice, in hindsight, would be to discuss with your loved one, when they are well, what they would want to happen if such an emergency arose.

The problems arise if you have *not* had these discussions and you are then second guessing at four o'clock in the morning what they would want.

I ended up signing the DNR order, and have subsequently lodged a DNR order with Mum's GP. This was not an easy decision, but after listening to the doctor at the hospital, and having a conversation with Mum's GP, I made an informed – albeit difficult – decision.

If you do lodge a DNR order with your loved one's GP, then they will give you a certificate. If one day you need to call an ambulance for your loved one, then if you hand the certificate over to the paramedics, they have to act on it.

Mum's DNR order is based around 'cardiac issues', but I believe you can get different DNR orders dependent upon your loved one's situation. How I see it, is it's about allowing a natural death, not a forced life with everything that that can be thrown at you and your loved one. But please, if you have time, do your own research. Try 'googling' DNR.

I sincerely hope you don't get asked this question at 4am, like I was, but I have nothing but praise for the doctors. Please don't be scared of discussing this issue with your loved one's GP; they will be so understanding. I felt really guilty asking Mum's GP for a DNR order after her stay in hospital, but he absolutely agreed with my decision given Mum's age and the 'life' she might have following a heart attack or other such event.

When making this decision, I put myself in Mum's shoes, and made the decision based on what I would want. That's the only real information I had to go on. I believe that if you go with 'what I would want', then you won't go far wrong.

I went back to Frimley Park Hospital later that afternoon and was informed that the operation had gone extremely well, but Mum had to stay in hospital for a couple of weeks and would also require physiotherapy for about a month.

Up until the fall, as I mentioned earlier, Mum was as fit as a fiddle for a 90 year old. But after the fall and operation, Mum suddenly had full-blown dementia – I know this must have been a shock to her, and it totally blew me away. I just couldn't get my head around what had happened, and indeed why it was all happening so suddenly.

Rapid onset dementia can happen after a shock, accident or other such event; I hadn't heard of it before, as I had wrongly believed that dementia came on slowly – not overnight!

Hospital tips

Hospitals by their very nature are noisy places and your loved one might get extremely upset by the people and hustle and bustle of the ward. People with dementia are usually extremely confused and upset; but even more so than usual in a hospital!

Part of my success strategy was to keep everything as normal as possible. But being admitted into hospital is anything but 'normal' and certainly not calm, which is key to keeping Mum content. Mum wouldn't eat the food they gave her; she only wanted my food and I had to be with her before she would eat it! This was a pretty tiring and upsetting few weeks for everyone concerned.

The nursing staff were all exceptional. I love the NHS, but unfortunately the staff are under so much pressure. Through no fault of their own, staff don't have a long time to spend with each patient. This is where you can help.

I didn't know that I could take Mum out of the ward until around day nine. A nurse suggested I take Mum for a 'walk' in the wheelchair. I wish I had known this from the outset as sitting next to a hospital bed for eight hours a day is not fun!

Wherever possible, please check with the nursing staff first. Make sure you get a wheelchair (if needed), or if your loved one is able to walk, take them outside for some fresh air or to the canteen and let them choose a nice hot drink of some sort – whatever they want.

This is me is a document that lets friends, carers and anyone looking after your loved one know all about them. *This is me* is particularly useful for hospital staff to understand their likes and dislikes and any problems your loved one has. This includes dementia, but also things like their eyesight, hearing and the medication they take.

If you haven't already got this document and completed it, then please do so, prior to anything happening! Here is the link: www.alzheimers.org.uk/get-support/publications-factsheets/this-is-me. Alternatively, please ask the ward sister for a copy of the form, or indeed ask PALS (Patient Advice & Liaison Service) in the hospital.

Have you heard of a Carer's Passport? Most hospitals have them. Make sure you apply for yours. A Carer's Passport, for dementia patients and carers, will allow you to visit any time of day or night to support your loved one. Some hospitals give you reduced parking fees as well. Please contact either your ward sister or PALS in the hospital for full information.

Mum used to get really down when she was bored and 'feeling useless'. Ensure your loved one is engaged and can get out and about. I found that chatting with Mum usually distracted her.

Make friends with the staff by being helpful and not getting in their way. I also found that buying the staff a box of biscuits or two always went down a treat. Talk to them and ask them what you could do for your loved one that would make their lives easier and your loved one less bored.

Audio books are a good idea. However, check if the sound is better with or without hearing aids in (if applicable). I know that when Mum is on the phone, she hears better without her hearing aids in. It's weird I know, but it's just one of those things I've learnt along the way.

I know that most hospitals have TV (paid for) but Mum got very confused and upset when she tried to get it to work and the headphones constantly got in her way. I eventually gave that up as a bad job.

Take in some photographs of your family or friends. This will help your loved one feel as though they are not quite so isolated and alone; they can get very upset at times. Having photographs means they'll have something that is familiar to them.

Meal times

Patients are normally given a menu the day before to choose what meals they would like. Mum's reading ability at this point was pretty non-existent.

A word of advice: before you leave for the day, please ask one of the care assistants to give you a menu before you go, so that you can complete the menu form for your loved one. I found that Mum just 'went with the flow' and said yes to anything they suggested. No wonder she wouldn't eat the food; she didn't order anything she liked. You know your loved one better than anyone else. That's another good reason why you should complete the *This is me* form.

Being talked about!

None of us like being 'talked about', particularly when we are in the same room! This is true in any situation where there are two or more people with your loved one. Sometimes you might have to give your friends, family and even doctors and nurses a gentle reminder that your loved one is also in the room.

Most people do speak directly to your loved one, or at least 'share the conversation', but occasionally people do forget at times. It really upset Mum when people did this to her, especially when they were talking about her! Remember that although your loved one might have dementia, they are neither deaf nor dumb and are definitely not invisible.

Mum did get somewhat cross one day with a very young GP (well, they all look young to me! A bit like policemen!). She calmly said to him that it would be respectful if he could talk to her and *not* about her with others! I don't think that young doctor will make the same mistake again in a hurry.

Mum is great on a one-to-one basis when having a conversation, but she gets very muddled when two or more strangers (for example, doctors) are with her and all talking at once. So if you can avoid this scenario, it will save you a lot of angst.

CHAPTER 4

CARE(LESS) HOMES!

After two weeks in hospital, Mum went back to her own home, with the assistance of carers coming in twice a day and Meals on Wheels popping in at lunchtime. The carers were kindly provided by the NHS and I organised Meals on Wheels through a local charity run by volunteers; the lunch cost about £5 a day.

I then spent weeks running backwards and forwards with food, love and doctor's and consultant appointments. I'm not sure who was more exhausted, Mum with the side effects of a fall, dementia, anaesthetic, operation and little sleep in the hospital as someone snored all night, or me!

Interestingly, Mum never could remember why she fell in the first place; she hadn't tripped. Given what I know now, I believe that she had a mini stroke, called a transient ischaemic attack (TIA). It wasn't apparent at first, because she was muddled after the operation and I put it down to the hospital environment.

Mum rapidly lost her confidence and went from being totally independent to becoming extremely reliant on me. She now felt 'nervous' about being on her own. This was something that I'd never experienced before with Mum; it was a huge shock to me and her.

I know I panicked at this stage, but if I had just taken a step back and breathed, and googled a lot, not to mention seeking help from her GP, I believe they could have offered me help. But not knowing the questions to ask is a real stumbling block.

The carers left after six weeks, and the physio signed her off as 'fit' (well, as much as she could be) after two months. However, Mum's insecurities grew worse. I had hoped that this would be a passing phase, but sadly that wasn't to be the case.

At the beginning of June 2015, Mum started to deteriorate further. She started to fall over again and was 'out of sorts'. I had to do something; but what?

I decided to put Mum into a care home for two weeks of respite care so that I could have a break and work out what to do for the best. Whilst she was in the care home (which she absolutely hated), I started to notice that she really wasn't well.

Unfortunately, due to the lack of care and staff at the care home, she became doubly incontinent – they put her in 'nappies' and told her to just wee and poo into her 'pad'! I won't name the care home, but they do have an 'Outstanding' rating!

A few days later, I noticed that Mum's face was very red. The care home said she had sunburn. But how could it be sunburn when she hardly left her room? It turned out that Mum had 'low sodium' thanks to all the pills she was on, following her hip operation.

I called an ambulance and she was admitted to hospital. The next day whilst I was with her, on my birthday, she had a seizure thanks to the medication. I'd never seen anyone have a seizure before and it was *so* scary. I screamed and got the attention I was looking for.

When I shouted 'HELP', doctors and nurses appeared within seconds. It seemed like they were coming through the walls once the nurse pressed the Red Panic Button. At least five doctors and three nurses surrounded her bed. I was 'got out of the way' and was 'looked after' by the lovely visitors in the ward.

Mum was immediately taken for a brain scan, but no damage 'appeared' to have been caused. I didn't believe that. Well, that was a birthday to remember – Happy Birthday to me!

Huge kudos again to Frimley Park Hospital. The staff, doctors and nurses could not have been more caring.

Tips when looking for care homes

There is an awful lot of advice out there about choosing the right care home. Care homes spend millions of pounds advertising their services. In my humble opinion, it is the staff, whom they pay peanuts to, who either make or break a care home.

When doing research for a suitable care home for your loved one, these are the things I think you need to consider and be aware of.

Some of the homes have very glossy brochures. When you're shown around, everything looks 'glitzy' and glamorous. This was the case with most of the ones I looked at. They show you round, you get to see the day/communal lounges for socialising, the smart dining room and inviting menus, the activities board (or is that 'bored'), a sample bedroom where residents have their own TV and en-suite bathroom with all the 'bells and whistles', but please dig deeper.

Do pop into the care home unannounced, for several different visits at different times of the day. Maybe take a quick picture with your phone of the menus and activities on the noticeboard. The first warning sign is if you get a frosty reception when you visit, with the staff saying that they weren't expecting you – especially after your third unannounced visit!

Do visit during meal times to see how much help the residents are given and how tasty and easy to eat the food is. Steak and jacket potato might sound delicious, but how many of the elderly folk can actually cut up and chew their meat?

Perhaps Italian or something with olives and herbs is not ideal for a 90 year old? That's my opinion anyway. I think giving residents a choice, like an omelette, fish and chips, cottage pie – good 'old-fashioned' food – is far more the order of the day. It's easy to eat and tasty. These are the foods they remember from a time before they got dementia or became frail.

For me, it's more about their dignity – being able to feed themselves and actually enjoy their meals, which is often the highlight of their day. Good old fish and chips, or sausages and mash; tasty and nutritious.

Do arrive during an activity and watch what they do. How engaged are the residents and the activities leader?

Do check out the day rooms and see how many of the residents are in there chatting away – I bet very few.

Do speak to as many staff as you can, preferably when the person showing you around is not loitering around you. See if the carers speak clearly, in an audible fashion, and ask them questions about what they love about being a carer.

Do have a quick glance in as you go past the bedrooms. Count how many of the residents are just sitting in their rooms or in bed watching TV.

Do your research on salaries! You can find out on the internet how much money the staff are paid, compared to the fees people are paying! Try www.gumtree.com – if you type in the search box 'Carers wanted' you can then see how much they are likely to be paid.

Do ask the person who is showing you around about the turnover of staff. If they haven't got the information to hand, then ask them to send it to you. To be honest, if they say they don't know, then alarm bells should start ringing. The turnover number will tell you an awful lot; not just about how the staff are treated but also about the care that your loved one will receive. If the staff aren't happy, that will rub off on the residents!

After three or four visits, you should have an idea of how frosty or friendly your reception is. Do *not* only visit once – although everything might seem excellent, it's *not* about the presentation!

In my opinion, some of the less modern care homes, with more 'lived-in' furniture and fittings, seem to have a far better 'homely' feel. It's not all about the shiny leather and modern furniture. The residents are likely to be 80+ years old, and have furniture that they love and are as comfortable as a second skin.

Do make sure you check out the care home's menus and activities. They are likely to be far more suited to the elderly than those rather modern menus you find in the rather 'swanky, yet austere and new' buildings that appear 'perfect'.

It must be said, I do enjoy a five-star hotel for a weekend break; however, I love going back to my cosy and comfortable home. Do think about your loved one's care in the longer term – it's not just a weekend break! To put this into context, I once lived in a four-star hotel with work for a year. Yes, the first few weeks were fine, but then I started to discover the cracks and the staff started to see you as their friend and confide in you. I started to see and hear all the faults and it became claustrophobic for me. I would far rather be in a cosy B&B long term with lots of cheery faces around me.

Once, whilst wandering around a potential care home for Mum, I came across an acquaintance, whom I had met several times over the past few years. I had no idea that her Mum was either in a care home or so poorly.

I stopped to say hello and began to have a chat with her, much to the disgust of the lady showing me around! My friend offered me a cup of tea. She told me an awful lot about the home and that the only reason she and her Mum 'suffered' it was because it was the only place that had the facilities to look after her Mum. This is despite this care home also having a 5* 'Outstanding' rating.

One thing I am sure of though is that there is a care home to suit everyone; the problem is finding the right one for your loved one. That's the tricky bit!

I appreciate that *no* care home is perfect, but you really need to do your homework thoroughly and not be swayed by looks alone. I guess that goes for anything in life.

CHAPTER 5

CARERS AT HOME

After Mum's seizure, given the 'care' Mum had received in the 'Outstanding' care home, I realised that:

a) Mum wasn't ready to 'live' in a care home, but also

b) Mum couldn't live independently any more, and

c) My home wasn't Mum-friendly yet, given her inability now to walk up or down stairs safely.

So, in June 2015 whilst Mum was in the care home I decided that she needed a live-in carer. I managed to organise this within a week of her being home (I stayed with her in the interim). I contacted a live-in care agency, in a bit of a panic! I was never advised – I had to just react and do what seemed right.

I found what 'appeared' to be a fab agency who provided live-in carers and felt that I had fallen on my feet. They were a small independent agency and the ladies were lovely. The company sent over 'Suzi' (names have been changed) and she seemed perfect. To be fair to Suzi, she was good. I always knew she was 'short term' as she had another contract lined up and anyone can put up a good front for a couple of months.

Suzi was with us for two months. She was fun and kept Mum going. She kept her interested and fed, warm and mainly cared for. I popped over daily to give Suzi her two hours off every day. This meant at least three hours out of my day, seven days a week, was spent travelling to and fro, doing shopping, and taking Mum to GP appointments, the dentist etc.

The next couple of carers were 'OK' and things seemed to be working out, with me covering for the carers for two hours a day and at GP and dental and hospital appointments. The live-in care cost around £4K a month, and I spent around 30 hours a week with Mum whilst working full time and trying to 'have a life' too (ha ha).

However, the lovely small agency was swallowed up by a larger company. Things quickly changed, and we were 'given' a new carer who seemed to know best!

(I guess that's what happens in today's world. If you have something good, then someone else wants it and sometimes spoils it. Is that called 'progress'? Here come the 'glossy brochures' again! Am I getting cynical, or am I already? I found the glossier the brochures, the more I doubted the company; isn't hindsight and age a wonderful thing?)

The carers 'appeared' to care, but Mum started to lose weight and had a lot of UTIs (urinary tract infections – see Chapter 9 for more information).

I mention being 'given' a carer above, as that's what happens. The agency say they 'match' the carer with the family and your loved one. Really? *Wrong!* They give you whoever they happen to have available on their books at the time. Please don't be fooled.

Yet again, I'm only sharing with you *my* experience. I'm sure that this doesn't happen all the time, or does it?

Unfortunately, the next carer couldn't cook English food. I bought her several 'easy-to-cook' books but I think they were too complicated for her. Whether it was the written English that she couldn't comprehend, I just don't know.

It became clear that the carer had never cared for anyone before. She'd apparently been on a carer's course for a week, where she was apparently taught how to cook and care for the elderly.

I continued going back and forth to Mum's house to cover for the carer for two hours every day. I began to get tired – there were more visits back and forth to the GP's with various UTIs. I noticed Mum's health deteriorating daily and she was seriously losing weight. She was now a size 8 and 7 stone. She became more and more needy and only wanted me.

When I wasn't with her, I was getting about 20 phone calls a day asking when I was going to visit her as she hadn't seen me for weeks, and she was getting very panicky.

Real alarm bells then started to ring. Mum was losing weight, having UTIs every other week, confusion and weakness reigned, and her eyes were sad and tired. These are not good signs. But I felt like I was a rabbit caught in the headlights. Instead of 'stepping back', I just felt that I was reacting to every little thing. However, you do also to have to have the patience of a saint.

Mum used to go to the day centre twice a week, thank goodness. She went under *huge* protest and I had a terrible time with her beforehand and afterwards, but she was always fine when she got there.

I phoned my lovely friend Tina, and I was telling her my woes as I knew she would understand. She was a fabulous listener and at the end she said, 'My Mum used to be a carer; would you like me to speak to her to see if she can help you out?'

To cut a long story short, out went the 'carer' and in came Tina's Mum, Diane. And, breathe!

The change in Mum was almost instantaneous – good food, good care, love and kindness; I can never thank Tina and Diane enough. Unfortunately, I knew that this wasn't a long-term solution as Diane had literally put her life on hold to come and help me out. At this point, I decided that Mum was going to come and live with me.

Given that Mum had taken to 'straying' (trying to escape the confines of her flat when the carer was with her at 3am) and her walking was not great, I knew that she needed a bedroom on the ground floor. Although Mum's 'straying' stopped the minute that Diane arrived; make of that what you will!

I thought about a stair lift, but if Mum woke in the night and went wandering, or to the loo, even with a stair gate, I think she might've fallen over it and tumbled to the bottom of the stairs. So this was not an option.

Building work then started in earnest to my home. I converted my integral garage into a bedroom with an en-suite bathroom for Mum. Diane was an absolute pillar of strength throughout and stayed with Mum until the garage was finally converted.

Diane is now one of my 'back-up' carers and takes over from me when I go away for a few days at a time. I still have carers in to look after the 'care' needs of Mum, but I trust Diane implicitly. I would urge you to find a 'Diane' as you will need her; please ask friends, family and acquaintances for recommendations as they can be a lifesaver.

The carer (Claire) I have for Mum has been with us for a year and a half now.

CHAPTER 6

CHOOSING THE RIGHT CARER FOR YOUR LOVED ONE

So where do you find good-quality caring help?

This is so hard to answer. I got lucky eventually with our lovely Claire. However, I learnt many lessons before I finally struck gold!

Firstly, check with your council about their care provision and what your loved one is entitled to receive. Or, again, visit Age UK.

In order to be heard, screaming and getting angry is unfortunately part of a carer's lot – as nobody seems to take the blindest bit of notice of you unless you 'throw your toys out of the pram'. Why should this be the case? Well, it shouldn't and by my very nature, this totally goes against the grain.

You will need to put your 'business hat' on to fight for your relative or friend. Nothing comes easy and nobody tells you what help is available, or more commonly, what help is *not* available. Sad but true, there is *zero* money in social care and if you think there is, then please think again.

My experience is that you get pigeon-holed and 'put into the system' of various care organisations.

You are assigned a social worker who comes to see you, makes promises that they can't keep, and then you don't hear anything from them again. Just a heads up, please don't be disappointed if this happens to you. Don't pin your hopes on what they promise, because in my experience, it just does *not* happen, even if they say you will be fast-tracked as a priority. All I can say is I am still waiting, four years later, and I haven't heard so much as a dickie bird from anyone. Yet another 'hey ho' moment or is that an 'aha' moment? I don't blame the social services department at all; it's just that their hands are tied. In my honest opinion, if you don't expect anything then you won't be disappointed.

I didn't really know where to go when I started out, and to be honest I thought I would just need help for an hour in the morning and 30 minutes at night. How wrong I was.

Trying to juggle a full-time job (even though I am self-employed – see Chapter 11 for more on this) and running a home, trying to have a life etc. is absolutely impossible when you are caring for someone with dementia. I would often end up crying from sheer frustration and exhaustion.

My first port of call was to look on Gumtree for a part-time carer. Please don't ask me why, but I really didn't know where else to start. Because social services 'daren't' offer you practical advice, you really are left to your own devices. I am guessing it's the 'sue' culture of the UK that means that nobody dare give you advice.

I got many responses to my advert on Gumtree, but one stood out. She didn't reply to my ad with the usual 'I'm caring, trustworthy, etc.'. She gave me advice on the 'Dos and Don'ts of employing a carer', including a suggestion that you shouldn't just employ one carer, but several. Always have a back-up plan!

She got the job. She actually had her own independent care company and employed five carers. She organised the diary and knew who was going to be turning up and when.

What I didn't do was ask for references – something I really should've done and would respectfully suggest you do, no matter how desperate you're feeling. And I was desperate! I needed help as quickly as possible, especially as Mum was still doubly incontinent thanks to the 'care home'.

Luckily for me, it worked out quite well for about eight months and Mum had three regular carers. They came in for an hour in the morning and for about 45 minutes in the evening.

Unfortunately for me, this lady's business grew rapidly. We started getting carers we didn't know. They didn't have definite time slots and so we never knew who was coming, or more importantly, when!

I was constantly having to change my business meetings around the carers and Mum grew crosser and crosser when they were late, as was I because I was experiencing huge pressure from Mum when she was upset. Time is a real issue with dementia patients and that's why routine and timings are so important for them.

Keeping Mum calm and in a routine, not to mention consistency of care, is paramount to both her welfare and mine. Can you relate?

At the end of the eight months I tried to remain calm. Having looked after Mum pretty much full time, I realised that if this continued then something would happen to me. I decided I needed someone for the whole morning and then again for 45 minutes in the evening.

This happened sooner than expected. One day I blew a 'head gasket' with the carer and gave her notice. I was at the end of my tether with the inconsistency of care and the timings and Mum getting cross with me for the carers not turning up on time. Not to mention the UTIs that Mum had started to get again on a regular basis. Unfortunately, you, as the main carer, will get it in the neck for everything that goes wrong – whether your fault or not. It's just the way it is and please try to have a thick skin as you are going to need one. It's not you, but your loved one will only feel 'safe' having a go at you, because they can!

As luck would have it, one of the carers who was looking after Mum had decided that she had also had enough of the company too. A perfect match was made and Claire started part time with us almost immediately.

I certainly don't recommend you losing your temper and firing the care company without a backup plan because you could find yourself entirely on your own. An even worse case scenario – unless you are good at changing 'nappies', cleaning teeth and are an expert in care of the elderly.

From the moment Claire came to look after her, Mum got better every day. No more UTIs. She started becoming more confident and was happier within herself. I was in a better place too because I could breathe and felt less stressed.

Today, Claire looks after us all. She does however still look after some of her other clients as she couldn't bear to let them down. I totally respect her for that.

Finding the right carer for you and your loved one is crucial to your survival. Here are my top tips:

- Does your loved one like them?
- Always ask for a reference – preferably three
- Check out their social media profiles to see what they are really like
- Are they good listeners and can they communicate clearly?

- What care qualifications do they have?
- Do they have their own insurance?
- Are they DBS (Disclosure and Barring Service) checked?
- Do they drive and have the necessary insurance?
- Do they have a happy disposition?

Don't just take their word for it. Ask for proof. Also, always keep your handbag hidden. I have always felt, rightly or wrongly, that I didn't want to act any differently than I did before I had carers in my home. But I believe that if you do leave a purse hanging around it could be just too much of a temptation. I am definitely not saying that I have had any money go missing as I haven't, but please do not put temptation in the way, however comfortable you feel. I am not saying that you shouldn't trust carers because 99.9% are totally trustworthy, and like I said earlier, 'one bad apple…', but the bottom line is that you are letting strangers into your home. You just need to be mindful, like you would with anyone coming to do any work in your house, from window cleaners and boiler service people to oven cleaners. I have always been really fortunate with all the carers and tradespersons I have ever employed, but I think it's always best to be safe rather than sorry and then there can never be any ill feeling or unease on either side.

From your point of view, make sure you write a list of all the things you want the carer to do – a job description. And make sure you can communicate with each other.

Claire does pretty much everything for us. Claire's job description would look something like this:

- Personal care for Mum
- Making appointments with the dentist etc. and taking Mum there
- Shopping
- Taking Mum out shopping, to garden centres, etc.
- Washing
- Ironing
- Cleaning
- Answering the phones
- Making meals
- Chatting with Mum about anything and everything
- Taking Mum to audiology appointments, etc.
- Taking Mum for walks
- Exercises for Mum

You will also need a Care Plan. A Care Plan is a document which clearly states what duties you expect of the carer. It will include:

- Their name and how they like to be addressed, Mr/Mrs or by their first name
- Their age and date of birth
- Home address

- Their GP's details – name, address and telephone number
- List of medications

This is followed by a paragraph outlining what you expect of the carer, whether they live with you or in their own home.

In another paragraph, say what is wrong with your loved one – dementia/Alzheimer's. I would also state here if they have problems with mobility and other issues like hearing aids, false teeth, etc.

The morning (AM) call and Bedtime call from the carers would look something like this, but obviously you can amend to suit your loved one. Also, you need to think of how long this call will take because if your loved one is anything like Mum, then she doesn't like to be hurried or rushed. So I would respectfully suggest an AM call would be 45 minutes to 1 hour and the Bedtime call would take approximately 30 minutes.

Again though I would stress that routine is so very important for their welfare, so a regular time and one carer is perfect. Mum has Claire during the week and Donna at the weekends and that works perfectly for all.

AM call

- Assist loved one into the bathroom and give them a shower or bath, or just a full body wash, whatever they prefer

- Wash hair – so many times a week
- Assist loved one out of the shower and dry and apply body cream to legs and dress with clothes of his or her choice

Bedtime call

- Assist loved one to the bathroom
- Wash, teeth brushed etc. and help them either to bed or into the living room; dependent on the timings
- Leave a cold drink and biscuits by their bed for the night-time
- Ensure that 'Careline' personal alarm is always worn

The above 'calls' are just an example. Any carer worth their salt will help you put a full Care Plan into place. But obviously if things improve or decline, then the Care Plan can be amended as appropriate.

Care Book

This is especially important if you have more than one carer. This book will contain any concerns a carer might have, and they can use it to mention any problems or concerns, or indeed anything positive that might have occurred during the day or night. This book will be available to all and any GP callouts etc. I actually use a large diary, which does the job very nicely.

Medications

To assist with medications, speak to your GP and pharmacist and they can organise a dosette box for your loved one's pills. The pharmacist will create this dosette box for you so you can just open up the box for the correct pills at certain times of day. So one less job for you to have to do.

Please have a list of medications, dosages and times and days available at all times, probably kept at the front of the Care Book. The Care Book should also include:

- A medical 'potted history' of problems, e.g. broken hip (how it was fixed)
- The DNR (Do Not Resuscitate) certificate, if appropriate
- And even more important is a list of allergies, e.g. Penicillin

Your loved one must feel safe and secure. Consistency of care, not to mention routine, daily activities and love, are the most important things you can give to someone with dementia. Along with good nutrition, whatever that may be, and lots and lots of liquid.

However, I would sincerely suggest that you don't put *all* your eggs in one basket. As my original carer said, always have a back-up plan. She is not wrong, however good your carer is, or indeed how comfortable you feel with them. This advice should be taken as a warning – I'd definitely recommend getting another carer as a back-up as soon as possible.

Thinking back, I believe the carer who had staff really shouldn't have taken me and Mum on! Their core business was looking after the elderly who lived on their own, who were just 'grateful' that somebody turned up at all!

Some care agencies now have technology that 'clocks them in and out', but of course you don't know what they do when they get there if you aren't there!

I did find one carer sitting on Mum's bed texting her friends, whilst Mum was still in the bathroom waiting to be dressed! But that was just one carer and I'm certainly not saying that they are all like that; you just have to be aware and keep your eyes and ears open.

I've found that the majority of carers are excellent and do a really fab job, often in difficult circumstances. They certainly deserve far more money and respect than I believe they receive today. I know that I certainly couldn't cope without them.

However, one bad apple can spoil the bunch!

But, and this is a pretty *big but*! Please try not to get overly friendly with the carers. I have made this mistake in the past and have come to regret this. The problem is that if you become too friendly then the line between employer and employee can get blurred and if you then have a disagreement, for whatever reason, you lose a friend and, even more importantly, a carer for your loved one! Then you end up down the river without a paddle!

It will be difficult not to have a friendly relationship with your carers, but please try not to rely on them completely, as you will *always* need a back-up plan at some stage. Trust me on this one: I won't go into details, but if you don't take this advice, it will end up in tears unfortunately. If you do find an excellent carer it will be *so* difficult not to befriend them. Be polite and friendly, yes, but do not give them a key to the door (always use a key safe) and definitely do *not* give them a credit card or pre-pay card for shopping. Always give them cash and ask for receipts and keep an accounts book, so you know what they are spending your hard-earned money on.

CHAPTER 7

ALZHEIMER'S AND VASCULAR DEMENTIA DIAGNOSIS

On 13 February 2016, Mum moved in with me, my partner and my two cats – Biscuit and Fudge. She loved telling everyone that she now lived in a garage!

Mum was still not 'right' and I knew that her moods, well-being and memory were deteriorating fast. We were referred to a dementia specialist and he did all sorts of 'tests' with her. Mum had a Mini-Mental State Examination (MMSE). This test measures short-term memory loss, orientation, communication and perception. Please ask your GP for a referral for a test if you are in any doubt.

On the day we got her results, Mum was with me, and the consultant calmly stated that not only did Mum have Alzheimer's disease but vascular dementia too and an MMSE score of 16 – moderate dementia.

The MMSE is a test that gives doctors an insight into a patient's short and medium-term memory. Mum never finished the test as she got bored and very frustrated as some of the questions can appear repetitive. Even I was struggling with the length of time the test takes to complete; it seemed to go on for an hour or two – and it did.

I had known ever since Mum had her fall that she had dementia. I thought it was just 'mild' though. Not that I knew anything about dementia before all this... I thought it was a 'gradual' thing – normally apparently it is, but not in all cases.

I was horrified when the specialist told us *in front of Mum*. I really was concerned that she would just break down in floods of tears or worse. However, I had nothing to worry about. Two minutes later, we were back in the car and Mum was chatting as though nothing had happened. That's because as far as she was concerned, nothing *had* happened. Mum's short-term memory was such that she really didn't remember a thing about the appointment. But I did!

All Mum was interested in was getting home as soon as possible and having a nice cup of tea. Phew!

Unfortunately, there are no magic pills for dementia sufferers. Mum was offered some cholinesterase inhibitors that can apparently help the dementia sufferer to function at a slightly higher level. However, some of the side effects include nausea, vomiting, constipation, headaches, cramps, sleepless nights and dizziness.

I decided against the medication for Mum. Knowing how sensitive she is to any medication, I couldn't bear the thought of her having to deal with all the side effects too.

Unfortunately, because I declined the drugs, all support from the Memory Clinic was taken away.

They kindly put me on a waiting list for a specialist dementia course that would help me understand and cope. And guess what? I'm still waiting...

The reason why I state above that I thought Mum just had mild dementia was that I really didn't know any different then. But this is what I was faced with:

Mum's dementia signs in early 2015

- She's very confused – about the time, and what to do next
- She doesn't know the month or day, whether it's day or night time
- She's started to forget my name and sometimes calls me 'Mother'
- She can't read or write any more
- She can't dress herself, she tries to put her nightie over her clothes, and can't put her trousers on
- She doesn't know the prime minister's name
- She is absolutely terrified of being left alone
- She is constantly trying to find me or the carers
- She is forgetting words for things
- She calls the TV a computer – very confused
- She has started to wander / roam – particularly in the early hours of the morning
- Loss of interest in seeing or even talking with her friends on the phone

- She doesn't know where she is sometimes (even when she is home)
- Keeps talking about her parents; she had never done this before
- She gazes a lot – as if elsewhere
- Her confidence has totally gone
- Lack of interest in self
- She needs her food cut up; she doesn't seem to be able to use a knife and fork any more
- Her handwriting is awful – not that she wants to write!

In addition to the above signs that I noticed, you might also notice some of the following issues:

- Struggling to remember things such as what they had for lunch
- They appear to struggle when there is a group of people all talking
- They can't remember where their clothes are kept or where they put something
- Repeating themselves or cannot find the correct word for something
- Feeling confused and disorientated even in a familiar place
- Mood changes

I am certain that there are many other 'signs', but these are what I experienced in the early days. If in doubt, please go and see your GP; they might not know all the answers, but they are an excellent first line of support.

CHAPTER 8

GADGETS FOR THE HOME

To be honest, I had no idea of the type of gadgets or home improvements that I would need for Mum. It has been a huge learning curve over the years; and the gadgets and home improvements have changed over time. I have wasted huge amounts of money on buying 'stuff' that was a total waste of time.

However, the one thing I would very highly recommend is an alarm around their neck or wrist. Mum's fall on a cold kitchen floor with no-one near could have been fatal. Also, one of my Mum's oldest friends, Joy, fell in her garden back in November 2018 and she spent 24 hours alone and cold. Joy was subsequently alright, but she is now living in a care home as her daughters were just too scared that something similar might happen again, especially as Joy had sadly refused an alarm. I give below some other ideas for gadgets and equipment that should help to make the home a safer and more accessible space for a person living alone with a diagnosis of dementia.

Key safe

I strongly suggest having a key safe fitted. A key safe is a small metal box that is fitted to the outside of the house on the wall. A spare key is kept inside the key safe. Make sure your combination code is written down and kept in a safe place. You'll need to give it to people who need to gain access to your loved one's home, like their good neighbours.

Cameras

After Mum's fall I made the decision to put cameras in her flat. In the event of her ever having another fall, after the dreaded 9pm Sunday phone call, I would be able to open the app on my phone and see what had happened to her and where she was.

There is nothing more terrifying than getting a phone call to tell you that your Mum is in distress, and not knowing how or why and what you're about to walk into.

I did inform all the carers and social services that I had these cameras for Mum's safety. They were all very supportive of this. However, I would've been concerned if they hadn't been!

Mum was a bit upset at first about the cameras going up, but once she knew where they were fitted and where they were positioned (in her living room, hall, bedroom and kitchen) then she was happy that I felt assured she was safe.

If you are looking for cameras to be fitted, they start from around £20. Go onto Google, type in 'home cameras' and there are many pages to choose from.

Clock

To help Mum try to remember the day and time, I bought her a large digital clock, which clearly spells out the full day of the week, month and date in large bold letters. In fact, I have two – one in her bedroom and the other in the lounge – so she can easily see the day and time. It makes her feel 'less useless' too, knowing the day. It really is the little things that make a difference to their health and well-being. Please google 'large digital clocks for those with dementia'.

Bed bars

When I initially mentioned 'bed bars' to Mum, she immediately shut up shop and said 'No!' She had been having some small falls off the bed and I was worried, not to mention 'squashed' on occasions.

Mum had the idea that I meant those long and high bed bars, similar to those on hospital beds, so I showed her what I meant: about 18" high and 12" long, just big enough to stop her rolling out of bed and also something to hold onto when getting in and out of bed – Mum hasn't fallen off the bed since we got some and she also feels more secure; happy days.

Emergency alarms

I subscribe to Age UK's emergency alarm – www.ageuk.org.uk/products/independent-living/personal-alarm. That was a lifesaver for Mum.

You can also purchase motion mats to let you know if your loved one gets up in the night or tries to leave the home.

Door locks

When Mum was 'wandering' four years ago, I was faced with a bit of a dilemma: if I locked her in the house, for her safety, then she couldn't get out of the house. But should there be a fire, then she couldn't escape! Also, you could be accused of 'slavery' if you lock them in. I guess you can't win on occasion.

So I kept the key in the lock, which Mum was able to open – with a lot of practice. Luckily, after Mum came home to me, she didn't wander at all and hasn't since. Again, it's about keeping her safe and secure, and if she feels calm and loved then she has no need to wander.

Free-standing toilet frame

This is an absolute necessity, as it allows Mum to feel safe getting up and down. Thanks to the NHS who provided this for us.

Coloured toilet seat

Mum hasn't got one of these yet, but I do know we will need one in the future. She occasionally gets confused about 'where to go' and if she can see the brightly coloured loo seat, this will help with recognition.

Walking frames

Mum has several now, actually more, but she just uses two: a Zimmer and a three-wheeled rollator. Mum uses the good old traditional Zimmer once she goes to bed, as it is solid and safe, especially if she needs to get up in the middle of the night and is a little woozy.

During the day she uses a three-wheeler, with a little tray and basket. It's very easy to wheel and is a lot lighter than the Zimmer. Mum's is purple! A three-wheeled folding rollator.

She did try out a couple of four-wheeled rollators with a seat, but unfortunately these were just a bit too cumbersome for Mum; she's only about 4'10" and 8 stone now, so fairly tiny – which has its uses at times, especially on the odd occasion when she has fallen on me (in slow motion)!

Wheelchair

I bought Mum a bright pink wheelchair! Pink is my favourite colour and to start with she wasn't too impressed, but when people started chatting with her and smiling because they hadn't seen a pink wheelchair before, it made her happy.

The receptionists at the doctor's, hospitals, etc. always remember her too, and smile. Mum loves it when people smile at her; it makes her feel good about herself. Another win-win.

One tip is to try to buy the lightest one you can; but this is obviously dependent upon the size of your loved one. To be honest though, I don't find even the lightest one that light, but maybe I'm just an unfit wimp? It's more about the handling of them, than the weight!

And don't forget a wheelchair cushion to make it more comfortable. Mum has a problem with her lower back and we use a Union Jack beanbag which seems to help. I bought it at a service station when Mum was in a lot of pain on a motorway journey and it's lasted four years so far! Cheap and cheerful and does the trick.

I actually had to change my car to accommodate Mum and her wheelchair. A neighbour once said to me, 'But what's happened to your convertible?' Sadly it just wasn't practical, and in any case, how often do you get to put the roof down in the UK anyway? I'm happy, 'keeping up with the Joneses' is just not important to me any more. If a car is easy for Mum to get in and out of and accommodates everything she needs, then I'm content.

Shower seats and rails

I would highly recommend hand rails around the house; if you would like help with where to position these, then please contact your GP who will be able to get you a referral with the physio outpatients department at the hospital. They will come around to your home and even fit them in the right place and at the right height for your loved one. I guess that you will have to check with your local hospital for this though; but we got lucky.

I purchased and had fitted a fixed shower seat for Mum; they are far stronger than a little free-standing seat. Again, 'security' is key to their well-being. Unfortunately, after Mum's two-week stay in a care home, she has adamantly refused to have a shower since. Some you win...

Cordless kettle tipper

I did buy one of these and also a small 'travel' kettle, but it soon became apparent that neither were 'safe' for Mum. I do believe that these are brilliant for the disabled, but Mum's co-ordination, together with her trying to 'hang on to' her Zimmer frame, just wasn't conducive to making a safe cup of tea. But a fab idea though.

I was trying to make Mum as independent as possible, but I think I will stick with the job of 'tea-towel folding' and simple things that make her feel useful without the danger of scalding or hurting herself.

For more gadgets and ideas for the home, please visit www.alzheimers.org.uk

CHAPTER 9

THINGS I'VE LEARNT

Having Mum live with us is like having a newborn, or more accurately, a toddler: you daren't leave them alone, un-safeguarded, for a minute.

Mum, luckily for me, isn't so much a danger to herself, but she panics if alone. That must be so frightening for her, especially if she has forgotten where she is.

I seem to have been fortunate enough to have missed out on Mum turning on the gas and forgetting, or putting cat food in the fridge, plus all those awful and potentially life-threatening events. So I'm grateful for that, but we did go from 99% 'normal', whatever that is, to moderate dementia overnight, so action had to be taken really quickly.

What I will say is that if you 'suspect' that something is wrong, then get it checked out as soon as possible by your GP. Your 'gut' instinct does not lie to you and please don't be fobbed off, or else worse things will follow. Even if your gut instinct is wrong, it's best to get things checked out really quickly, or else they can deteriorate quite quickly. And it's a good idea to put your own mind at rest, as you have enough to worry about.

Signs that I tend to keep an eye on are:

- Appetite/weight – it's a good idea to weigh your loved one once a month
- Temperature
- Constipation – which can cause confusion
- UTIs – even more confusion
- Disorientation – even more than normal
- Incontinence – which is unusual for them
- Sleeping more than normal during the day

I have got to say that at my doctor's surgery, Hill-view Medical Centre (HMC) in Woking, Mum has had the very best of care possible. Special thanks must go to Dr Natasha Shah who has been a true pillar of strength: she listens, is caring, supportive and a true professional to boot – I feel blessed having her on our side. She's so kind to both of us and totally 'gets' our situation, and talks and listens to Mum and gives her time with dignity. The NHS at their very best once again. Thank you so much to all the doctors, nurses and support staff at HMC for all your support and understanding at all times.

Relationships and Mum

You won't realise at first how caring for your loved one *will* have an impact on *all* your relationships, in life and business. If you have taken on the caring role for a loved one then this will affect everything in your life, for better and for worse.

If you pay too much attention to your children, partner or friends, your loved one will get upset and if it's the other way around you end up having *everybody* upset at you. But you do need time for your family, friends and partner and you need to make time. Easier said than done however.

This is where good neighbours and carers come in. You need nights out with your family, friends or partner and to have some fun; because if you don't, you will lose it altogether – your identity, self-worth and so much more. It's not worth it and it will not do you or your loved one any good.

Try to take short holidays away together. I appreciate that this isn't always possible and can be financially restrictive, especially if you are paying someone to care for your loved one and are having to pay out for accommodation too!

But if you know a friend is going away for a few days, offer to 'house sit' and just spend some quality time with your family, friends or partner; it doesn't even matter if it's just 'down the road', but you do need some time off or else you will end up going bananas too!

Also, your GP may well have a Carers' Respite Fund. This is approximately £300, which will give you and your family, friends or partner some time alone, and allow you to pay a carer for a few days to take care of your loved one whilst you take a couple of long-earned days off. Please don't be afraid to ask for this help; that's what it's there for. You might have to fill in a form again, but I guess that's a carer's lot.

There is no doubt about it that whatever you 'try' and do to keep your relationships on track, you are going to hit some hurdles. Please try to remember that your friends and family have not changed, but *you* have. And they are finding it hard to come to terms with it all too. But unfortunately, unless you are Super Woman, or Man, you will fall down on occasions and with all the demands from everyone to everything, you can't do it all. I know you will probably want to, but that's when cracks start to appear.

I'm guessing, but obviously don't know, that a husband might feel somewhat neglected to start with when his wife has a newborn. His wife's attention, quite rightly and naturally, will be focused on the baby and not the husband, especially to start with.

One thing that Mum absolutely hated at the start of our journey, and to a lesser extent now, is if I was outside having a chat with a friend. I think she thought we were 'conspiring against her' or other such thoughts; but that's the disease talking, not Mum.

If you try to put your loved one's 'hat on', then it will be far easier to understand why they can get so upset over trivial events. But trivial events to you and me can be *mountains* to your loved one with dementia as everything becomes exaggerated.

Yes, of course I speak to my friends about Mum, but just to bounce around new ideas, and of course when I'm struggling to cope then a glass or two of Pinot Grigio and a giggle with my friends is definitely in order. But Mum has got used to that now; well, mostly!

That all said and done, you *do* need some time with your friends and loved ones and I do get, on occasion, told that I wrap Mum too much in cotton wool, but they don't really see the consequences of me not doing so! Even carers can also have a little dig at me, but I know it's because they care about me too – but sometimes you can't do right for doing wrong.

There are times though that I do know that Mum can do more for herself than she either lets on, or in practice would rather I do for her! Don't be fooled please and try to push them as much as they will let you.

I guess you have to strike a balance, but on occasion it involves walking a very fine line; at the end of the day, do whatever works for you. I'm a bit of a coward really; I would rather keep the peace with Mum – and on occasion 'tread on eggshells' with everybody else. But that's not easy either!

'Things'

If you have a loved one with Alzheimer's, one of the traits I find is that they have 'things' that they like to have around them. Mum's 'things' are remote controls and her walking stick!

I often find myself scrabbling around the house for a TV remote, only to find several hidden in her bedroom. Please remember that this behaviour is the 'disease' not them, but I believe that this is Mum's security blanket, so I let it go and let her collect as many as she wants; and she often does! But funnily enough, she only likes the black ones! So I have had to swap her white telly and white remote for a black telly and a black remote. I don't understand it, but if it makes Mum feel good, then I am fine with that. Whatever makes your life calmer and easier.

Mum really likes to have her walking stick with her at night and she won't go to sleep without it by her side. Maybe this is because her bedroom is on the ground floor. But when she goes to the loo at night with her Zimmer frame, she tends to take her walking stick with her and this bashes into her leg.

To overcome her stick bashing her leg and causing bruising and cuts, I have bought some shin pads for her at night. I know this sounds excessive but please google 'shin pads for the elderly' and the results will highlight some lightweight shin pads. They have stopped the bruising for us.

Bedtime

Night-time rituals are also very important, so that your loved one can feel safe and secure, which is key to someone with dementia. Mum likes to go into a nice 'warm' bed with the curtains open just enough so that she can see the street light, together with a cup of tea, milk and a banana, plus sweets and biscuits at the side of her bed. If I look at it from Mum's point of view, it's that she has enough to eat and drink until morning comes. Happy days.

As an aside, I always keep her bedside light on and a light on in the bathroom; also, there's a little pink bell that says *Ring for Hugs*; it just makes her feel 'secure'.

Food and diet

The problem I think is that they believe that they've just eaten. I'm not a doctor but I think their tummy doesn't send signals to their brain any more. So you really need to be their 'tummy' for them.

Little and often has now become my philosophy! Main small meals, interspersed with cakes and fruit – but all nicely presented. Presentation is key and I find that little and often is the way to go with Mum as she hates large portions and won't even try the meal if it looks too big. But don't be surprised if they leave just a little; Mum always leaves just a little on her plate – but hey, we all have our own foibles.

Sometimes you feel like you are wasting your breath asking what food they would like to eat! But try to always give them a choice. Although for breakfast, there is no choice – Mum just loves her poached egg and toast, all delivered nicely on a plate – breakfast in bed.

I suggest you serve something appetising, something they like, and put it down in front of them. Mum's favourite food is salmon, mashed potatoes and a little veg (if she has to!) with good old parsley sauce. Easy to eat and tasty.

Also, she loves home-made potato, onion, leek and veg soup – an easy way to disguise the vegetables! Add in a couple of stock cubes, simmer for an hour and then puree. Job done.

Mum's other favourite is roast chicken, and especially if she gets a Yorkshire pudding. And sometimes as 'Salmon Surprise', she gets a Yorkshire pudding with that too; it lets her know that she is loved.

I always lay the table for Mum, with a knife, fork and spoon, plus serviette and salt and pepper. Although I do know that Mum prefers a spoon these days, I always like to give her a choice, so she is in control, well a bit anyway. And she does on occasion use a knife and fork too.

As much as I am able, I do try to organise meals with Mum. But sometimes it's hard, especially in the summer, what with BBQs and tending to eat much later at night.

Routine is *so* important to Mum, so meal times, getting up etc., all around her pills, are fairly regimented. If my partner gets home late and wants a lamb or beef BBQ, as an example, which is too chewy for Mum to eat, then it's difficult. But what I tend to do in these circumstances is to give Mum her meal at 'her' normal time and then add a sausage from the BBQ, so that she feels included and part of the family – which of course she is.

Routine

Routine is so important to anyone living with dementia. I would sincerely suggest that you try and get a routine going as soon as possible.

Our daily routine goes something like this:

0730	Pills and water/tea
0830	Breakfast
0930	Get washed and dressed (with help from the carer)
1100	A walk or visit to the garden centre/supermarket
1230	Lunch
1400	A walk or short trip out
1430	Small cake and tea
1700	Pills

1730	Change into nightwear
1800	Dinner
2000	Bed

And, of course, copious cups of tea and coffee!

Never wake up late! Always set the alarm, even if you *always* wake up at 7am! One day I woke up at 9am and spent the day 'catching up' with a somewhat confused and upset Mum.

If you work from home, set aside an hour to do something fun and let your loved one know what that is and when it will happen.

Tablets

Mum is on relatively few tablets these days – Vitamin D to keep her sunny disposition, VitaEyes for her macular degeneration, plus some pills for her bones and some to help her have a good night's sleep and for 'mood'.

Her main prescription is for thyroxine. Mum has had to take thyroxine ever since she was about 30 and the dose hasn't really changed over this time.

Unfortunately, Mum had a small fall and ended up in A&E again recently. Luckily nothing was broken this time but the fabulous NHS doctor said he wanted to find out 'why' Mum had fallen. God bless the NHS again.

A blood test was taken and it showed that Mum's thyroid was not behaving. They have since increased the dosage, over a month or two, and the difference in Mum is awesome – she's so much more awake and lively.

I should have known (hindsight is such a wonderful thing!). Mum was sleeping all the time at one point. I had taken her to see the nurse at the doctor's surgery, but she had very gently suggested that it could be something to do with her age! The problem was that the daily sleepiness happened and grew worse over about a year; it was so gradual that I hardly even noticed.

But if you are worried about your loved one's mood or sleeping patterns, I would respectfully suggest that a blood test about twice a year wouldn't be a bad idea; it's an especially good idea to get their thyroid level tested.

Temperature

I also believe that their body clock doesn't tell the brain when it's hot. Mum appears to always feel cold, even at 30 degrees.

This is hard to manage, because when they say they are cold, even though it's hot in the house, you need to just put a blanket on them. But being too hot can lead to heat rashes and dehydration too; just one other thing to think about.

Dehydration

Dehydration is a big problem – not to mention UTIs. Enemy number 1.

Many of the doctors and nurses I've spoken with have told me to get Mum to drink more water. Yes, I *do* know this. Have you tried asking a 93 year old to drink water that they don't like?!

You can try until the cows come home. I'm telling you now that *they won't*! No matter how much you beg and plead. They might have half a glass just to shut you up, but that will be it – *no more ever*.

So, give them what they want. If that's copious cups of tea, then at least it's a drink. When they constantly leave half a cup of tea, just give them a fresh cup. They don't leave the tea because they don't like it; they leave it because they've 'forgotten' about it. And when your partner gets cross about the waste, tell them why they do it.

The best way around this is to have a tray or table in front of them, not at the side, whilst they have a drink. If they can see it, they will drink it. But that's not always possible. If they need to go to the loo in a hurry, you may end up with upturned tables and tea!

Alternate one cup of tea with one glass of cranberry juice or water. Let's hope you are more successful with water than I am. Mum refuses to drink water. They can become somewhat stubborn to say the least.

Mum, back in 2015, started saying things like, 'If you want me to drink more that's fine. I will pee all over the place. Is that what you want?'

If your loved one says, 'It's my birthday today,' reply with, '*Wow*, happy birthday, have a great day. Shall we celebrate with a lovely cup of tea?' Leave the room. Bring back a cup of tea five minutes later.

Signs of a UTI (urinary tract infection)

The best sign of a UTI is *your* gut instinct! Sometimes the changes are so subtle that if you blink, you'll miss them. The first signs to look out for are mood changes (anxiety, confusion), weeing in inappropriate places and a slightly raised temperature. Also, the colour of the urine should be fairly clear; if its brown or orange, then you definitely have a problem brewing.

One thing I do, if I suspect a UTI, is take a urine sample down to the GP as soon as possible to have it tested and get the appropriate treatment as soon as possible. Please ask the GP or receptionist for some spare bottles, so you don't have to get some prior to taking a sample.

On the note of temperature taking – buy the cheapest and most basic of thermometers. I've tried every expensive gadget going and they are hard to read and calculate. I suggest using your bog-standard thermometer that you place under the tongue for a minute. Easy peasy.

Technology and I should be kept apart, especially when it comes to gadgets. The simpler something is to use, the better, especially in times of panic or distress. So *KISS* it! – *Keep It Simple, Stupid*. I now live by this mantra and I don't go too far wrong.

Constipation

However much you care for your loved one, constipation, especially in combination with UTIs, is really difficult to deal with and makes them even more confused than before.

I used to really struggle with Mum's constipation as it made her so upset and it was so difficult to deal with, but coconut oil seems to have done the trick.

Mum used to have porridge every morning, so it was easy to stir in a spoonful of coconut oil. But as she prefers egg on toast these days, I now give her one coconut oil tablet every day and the difference, overnight, works a treat. It basically 'oils' the internal organs, especially the bowel, and everything seems to flow far easier these days.

I believe that in the past I misdiagnosed some of Mum's UTIs; I think she was simply constipated.

Going to the loo

Mum tends to often leave it too late. The best way around this is to suggest that she might want to go to the loo about every two hours or so.

But I think the reason that Mum leaves it too late is because she doesn't want to miss out on things – whether I have a friend here, or she's watching her favourite programme, *Father Brown*, on the telly. Please try to reassure them that they won't miss out on anything and you can pause the TV.

Never, *never and never* go out without checking that they have been to the loo. Even for 5 minutes! One day we went off to Waitrose (10 mins down the road). We spent about 15 minutes putting coats on, shoes on, transferring from the wheelchair to the car. We got to Waitrose and she announced that she was 'desperate to have a wee'.

So back home we went. Half an hour later, we started back on our journey – déjà vu.

Walking/exercise

Mum's walking has become far more laboured. But I don't believe this has really got anything to do with her legs, as her core muscles are really good (thanks to the yoga and Pilates). But I believe it is her brain that is telling her that she can't walk.

So, unless your GP says otherwise, please keep up with gentle exercise and also walking as much as possible, but you will need to have a lot of enthusiasm, patience and persistence.

I have bought Mum an electrical foot/leg machine, but she does moan about it. That's why a hard skin and persistence pays off – in the end! If you can stick at it for about 10 minutes, three times a day, it will make a difference to keeping their leg muscles exercised with very little effort from them!

The problem is that if she gives up walking and using her legs, we will then need a frame to get her in and out of bed and into a chair, and to be honest I don't think my back will take the strain! If you do have a 'lift', then it is supposed to be operated by two trained operatives… But if you are on your own, then what do you do?

So I will continue to be 'bossy', as Mum says, and continue to persuade her to walk and use her legs.

Feeling useful!

There is nothing worse than feeling 'useless'. Please try to create things for your loved one to do. It's not always easy, but here are some suggestions.

Shopping

Before you go shopping, create a shopping list *together* and then when you are in the supermarket, give them the list to let you know what you need. Also, walk slowly around and let them choose what they would like too. The familiar packaging and smells will let them know what they would like and it brings back memories too.

However, shopping has its dangers! Mum has now lost her sense of tact! She shouted out quite loudly the other day, *'Wow* hasn't that lady over there in the red dress got a *huge* bottom!!' Luckily, the lady concerned gave Mum a little wink and a smile, but sometimes the outcomes are not always quite so positive! They have lost some of their inhibitions, which at times is quite trying! She even told Claire the other day, who is a size 10/12, that she looked pregnant in the jumper that she was wearing! Good job Claire has a good sense of humour and totally understands the situation, but be warned that people with dementia do tell it exactly how it is and be prepared for the odd embarrassing moment or two.

Gardening

If your loved one can't garden any more, then at least get them to choose the plants, or flowers, from the garden centre. They might not be able to actually 'plant' them, but they can tell you what plants will look good with others and they can 'supervise' you watering and pruning them.

I'm hopeless at gardening, but having Mum tell me 'what is what' really helps and if we both get it wrong, well… What the heck – have a laugh about it. Laughter really helps.

Try!

Try and get them to interact with others, as much as possible. Mum doesn't really like 'old' people; I think because it reminds her that she isn't young any more… and she certainly doesn't want a room full of people talking all at once. In this situation, they will just get very confused, scared and then agitated, which is to be avoided at all costs!

But we have five-year-old twins (a girl and a boy) who live opposite us and they love to come in and show Mum their latest toys, from bicycles to Halloween costumes, and Mum's eyes light up every time she sees them. They seem to have a 'special bond', please don't ask me how, but she listens and smiles and makes all the right noises, and they in return giggle and smile; it's so lovely to see. Maybe Mum remembers when Sarah and I were little? But she definitely engages more with them than anyone else!

I have tried Mum with 'large' jigsaw puzzles, memory books, easy crossword puzzles etc., but none seem to do the trick. I think she is scared of failing, so doesn't try. So I don't push it any more; it would be lovely if she would like to have a go – but failing doesn't make her feel good.

Feeling useful is so important to everyone; that's what makes us all feel good. If you can help someone, how does that make *you* feel? So please try to give them something that helps you, so you get another win-win.

This can involve you asking your loved one to fold up tea-towels, cut up some veg, or peel a potato, or even involve including them in creating a menu for the week.

No surprises!

Mum hates surprises. She likes to know what is going to happen throughout the day and when. She certainly doesn't like 'strangers' in the home, as it upsets her routine and security.

Our days are a bit like 'Groundhog Day'– however, that works for Mum. Please remember that their short-term memory is pretty much shot to pieces. However, Mum's memory has returned a bit. I'm not saying a lot, but it's definitely far better than it used to be.

Security

Security is a huge part of Mum's well-being. Security and routine go hand-in-hand. If Mum feels, safe, secure and loved, she is, in the main, happy. However, once something topples over, e.g. strangers in the house, or too much noise, maybe in a supermarket, or even at home (except for the TV), then you are going to have a problem on your hands.

Recently, I reminded Mum that she was going to meet three of her oldest friends the following afternoon. Helen, who was hosting, had arranged the event with Sandra and Vivienne. I thought Mum would be excited about seeing them – *wrong* (again). She was scared stiff.

She *was* looking forward to seeing them two weeks ago, but now that 'tomorrow' had come around so quickly, she was very anxious. Anyway, I threw my toys out of the pram, as did Mum.

Sometimes, you will get cross, as we are only human. But putting yourself in their shoes will help you so much more. I'm not saying that you won't get cross again, but it may help you.

I sorted out this issue with Mum by cancelling the event and sitting down and talking with her about her fears, so that I didn't make the same mistake again. Talking is really good, because they will tell you what they would like to do.

What you think will be fun for them may not be any more. It may feel more like an ordeal. Don't judge them; be a good listener. Please remember that communication is key.

On this note, dementia is not like a broken bone; it's a broken brain! So only part of the brain is working. You wouldn't tell someone with a broken leg to run around the block and get over themselves? Well, I hope not!

But by understanding the broken brain, you can start to understand the problems they are experiencing. If you think back – when you put your baby in the arms of a stranger, they were likely to cry because they were scared of the unfamiliarity. That's what I find with Mum – Strangers = Danger... So don't be surprised when they are rude to your friends. They are scared and out of their comfort zone. Their home is their safe place and if they feel that it is being invaded, they will 'kick off' and quite rightly too.

If you are expecting guests, although they may be few and far between these days, always explain to your loved one who is coming, why they are coming and, more importantly for them... when they will be leaving! And please don't tell them a time that you 'think' your guests will leave, add an extra hour. Because if you told your loved one that they would be leaving at 11.30am, then at 11.30am on the dot they will be feeling that it's time for them to go and if they haven't, then you have fibbed to them – which leads to them feeling scared and up-set.

They really don't like their small world being changed or invaded; they just cannot comprehend why they are upset. Routine, routine and routine is the order of the day if you would like some kind of normality. Whatever that might be!

Mum's weekend carer had to bring along her granddaughter with her recently. The granddaughter is two years old and loves playing games and listening to cartoons on her phone, not to mention wanting her Grandma's attention at all times.

Sadly, one morning it all became too much for Mum and she accused the carer of shouting at her. In the carer's defence, to get heard over her grand-daughter, her cartoons and Mum's TV turned up high, she probably did have to shout to be heard…

Unfortunately, the lovely weekend carer had sev-eral jobs to keep the roof over her kids' heads and worked night and day shifts far more often than she should, but needed the money. And that day I think was sadly just the 'icing on the cake'.

So Mum ended up being stressed out and the car-er handed in her notice in floods of tears. Of course, this was now another problem for me… How did that happen?

I used to be able to create problems of my own well enough! But sweeping up after others' issues is just now part of my life too.

So the search for a new weekend carer began. As I said earlier, always have a back-up plan. And luckily, yes I did, but I could have done without having to use my back-up plan. Now I had to get Mum used to a new carer, which to be honest felt like it was going to be a pain, but I also needed to find someone else to become an emergency carer. But luckily for me, Mum and Donna, our new weekend carer, both get on like a house on fire and all you hear from the bathroom is a lot of giggling and Mum doesn't now have to deal with a noisy two year old.

You will keep 'stumbling', whether through your own fault or 'life', and you just need to keep moving on.

Some days, however, you will feel alone and want to speak to someone who is in a similar situation. This is really important or else holding in your worries and frustrations will not be good for your health. I found new friends and carers online in a Facebook group, called *Dementia Carers Support Group UK*. This group is *so* supportive, because we are all in the same situation. And we all help each other. Why not join us?

People will always judge you

The other week I parked in a disabled bay with Mum in a supermarket car park. I got out of the car, got my handbag off the back seat and was walking around to the boot – to get Mum's wheelchair out. Three cars drove past me and the looks the drivers and passengers gave me were horrible. If they had waited another few seconds they would've seen me heaving her wheelchair out of the boot.

I presume they thought I was parking illegally. People are so quick to judge and life is difficult enough.

Sometimes others might believe that they have something useful to say. But please remember that you are the person who knows your loved one best and you are the expert when it comes to caring for them – so smile politely and feel free to completely ignore them if you know that their advice isn't right for you.

CHAPTER 10

THINGS TO DO AHEAD OF SCHEDULE

Here are some important things to think about sooner rather than later.

Data protection

This is so infuriating but I understand why it's necessary.

When you phone the GP or a utility supplier, bank etc., nobody wants to speak with *you* because you aren't the named person on their database! Get your loved one to write to the different companies (you might have to do it on their behalf and get them to sign the letter) and add you as the person to liaise with regarding any decisions that need to be made.

Some service providers will accept a phone call, if your loved one can coherently give them permission for you to speak on their behalf; others will require a letter. Do this as soon as possible – the sooner the better. This will make your life *so* much easier going forward.

Claiming benefits

In my experience to date, everything is a constant battle and you have to fight for everything! Time, money and anything else you need for your loved one.

However, as I mentioned earlier, Age UK are a great source of information, as is the Citizens Advice Bureau. However, unfortunately no one organisation has everything in one place, so you do have to do a bit of digging, but when the information is found it's really useful.

An old friend of mine who has subsequently passed away had a chat with me and said that she didn't receive any benefits even though she had terminal cancer!

Unfortunately, being the optimistic person she was, she filled her forms in when she was having a 'good' day. However, the problem was that 99% of the time she was having a 'bad' day. Some days, she couldn't get out of bed to go to the toilet. She didn't want the world to think she couldn't cope. Being brave didn't help her financially. In fact, it left her substantially short every month.

After we had a conversation, I convinced her to 'tell the truth' and she ended up getting an extra £600 per month from the government. You must leave pride out of the equation. If you need financial support, don't be afraid to ask.

This book is not about benefits and the frustrations that go with it, not to mention the very lengthy forms, but I highly recommend visiting the Age UK website (www.ageuk.co.uk) for information on benefits. I've researched many different sources and Age UK seem to be the best.

Wills

I often wonder, 'What would happen if I wasn't around any more? Who would do all the things I do for my Mum?'

At this point I would sincerely urge you to either revise your will or get one drawn up. Consider what would happen to your loved one if anything happened to you. What would you want to happen to your loved one? Care home? Carer at home or friend or relative?

Also, you do need to think of putting a power of attorney in place, should anything happen to you. For further information on this, please visit www.ageuk.co.uk – I do find the Age UK website invaluable for information and advice.

Things I used to do

Please forget about the phrase, 'I used to…' I used to socialise a lot more, go out to work and be in and out of the house all the time. Now I plan, plan and *plan*!

I don't go out any more and that's my fault – not Mum's fault. You can't just 'go out' as and when you feel like it. The good news is, if you *plan* ahead, you can make things work for you.

CHAPTER 11

EMPLOYMENT VS. SELF-EMPLOYMENT

As someone who was self-employed prior to finding myself in a caring role as well, I feel truly blessed. I don't think many employers would've allowed me to take time off for the following reasons:

- Because Mum was ill
- The carer was having a day off or was sick
- To attend doctors' appointments with Mum
- To go to hearing aid clinics due to Mum's broken hearing aids
- To go with Mum for eye tests
- To go with Mum for dental appointments
- To go with Mum for hospital appointments

The list is endless. When caring for others, you often need to take time off work at the last minute! If you throw children into the mix, you might find yourself having to juggle a lot more balls too.

Caring for someone changes everything – your relationship with your loved one, your partner, family and friends. The dynamics will change because you have to put your loved one first and everyone else has to take a back seat as a result. Unfortunately, the one person who will suffer the most (emotionally and physically) is *you*.

Day centres are closing down all over the country as government and councils are having to tighten their belts. That means that you can't just drop off your loved one at 8am and pick them up at 6pm, if you work full time. You might be lucky in your area. Please check out your council's website and google local day centres.

Becoming self-employed is not for everyone; I get that. However, it might end up being the only job you can do, especially with all the extra responsibilities that you find yourself taking on.

If you rely on your job, knowing that you get a salary at the end of every month, together with other benefits, I want to let you know that there are other options. Why not turn your passion into a profit? Do you love doing something; a hobby? Have you thought of starting your own business? Is there something that you're good at? Why not write a list and find other ways of how you could earn money, possibly by working from home?

Being self-employed is hard work. It's the hardest work I've ever had to do in my life. Keeping yourself motivated is the hardest job of all. Going from a job where you are surrounded by your colleagues, supported by your manager, given projects to complete with deadlines that need to be met, to working alone with no one telling you what to do is a big change. You might find yourself becoming a 'jack of all trades and master of none'. Here are some of the 'hats' you'll have to wear, especially if you don't have the money to outsource to others:

- Marketing manager
- Administration
- Accounts/book-keeping
- Sales
- Secretary
- Research assistant
- Motivator
- Social media expert
- Boss and cleaner!

These roles are an awful lot to take on, especially whilst caring for someone else as well.

When you are in business, make sure you are part of a business community network such as *Fabulous Networking*. Meeting other business owners will help you get clients and move your business further forward.

When going out to 'networking' meetings, remember that 'strangers are friends and colleagues that you haven't met yet'.

Types of jobs to think about, especially around what you used to do

If you were a secretary, then think about becoming a virtual secretary (working from home) to support other small businesses. There are virtual secretarial agencies out there that employ people to work from their own homes and in their own time.

If you were a book-keeper, or accountant, then maybe try to get a job working from home; I have found more companies being flexible in this way. And if you don't ask, you certainly don't get.

Hairdressing or beauty, you could certainly do from home. Set up a Facebook page and try advertising there or again on Gumtree, or even the old-fashioned way on your local newsagent's window.

You could also look into buying a franchise. A franchise is part of a larger branded company that has been tried and tested and you get the support from the franchisor, at a cost. However, some franchises cost from around £5,000. An example of a franchise is McDonald's. However, there are many smaller franchises from accountancy to vending machines, home care to IT, training and consultancy. Please take a look at www.franchisedirect.co.uk for some ideas and information on the type of franchises that are available.

There is a vast world out there for the self-employed, all mainly working from home. So get googling and do some research. And remember that this should be fun and bring you independence.

CHAPTER 12

ACCEPT YOU ARE NOT PERFECT!

We're only human after all. It's hard to accept, but it's the truth. You're not perfect but neither is your loved one!

It's a huge shock to the system when your Mum or loved one, whom you haven't lived with for 30 to 40 years, is suddenly 'in your space' and is with you 24/7. Hand on heart, caring for a loved one is not for the faint-hearted. They say that during our 'life cycle' we revert back to needing more care than that of a toddler. I totally agree. No one can prepare you for the hard work that lies ahead when looking after a loved one.

Suddenly your life is turned upside down, inside out and on some days, you don't know which way is up. The time, work and frustration that you experience is never-ending.

Often life throws you a curve ball. Just when you think you're getting your life back on track, your children have gone to uni and you can start doing the things that you want to do, you are presented with a situation that changes your life forever.

Even if you have six brothers and sisters, please don't expect them to help! If they see *you* as the carer they'll be really happy knowing that their parent is being well cared for, but they have their own lives to live! Yes, they are selfish – but 'lucky' them. They might turn up for a few hours once a month or so, but if you expect them to do more than that, you're likely to be disappointed and end up damaging your relationship with them.

If you don't have any expectations of your siblings, then you *won't* be disappointed. The less you expect of others, the less hurt you will experience, so save yourself the anger, frustration and all the emotions that go with it. You only end up hurting yourself.

This is a really hard lesson to learn. You will expect friends and family to rally around you, but the truth is, they won't. They may have the best intentions but like New Year's resolutions, they start well but end really quickly unfortunately.

There's no point getting cross with them as they will disappear faster than you can say 'Eureka' and you will, at some point, need them on your side.

Whenever and wherever possible, please keep the communication lines open. I know it's hard! Please be kind to yourself and others no matter how hard it appears to be at times. Don't expect them to show you any kind of recognition; they probably won't. Some might be feeling guilty enough as it is without saying it out loud.

They *do*, however, appreciate you! Why? Because you take all the stress, worry, guilt and burden away from them. Is this fair? Hell no, but that's life! You are not going to change others. The only person you can change is yourself.

Don't have any regrets. There will always be a negative voice in your head saying, 'You can do better.' Make your loved one's last years happy ones. Create special memories together and if you can, take lots of photos. Always remember you are doing the best you can with the resources you have.

Life is not going to be easy at times. I'm the first to admit I'm no angel, nor do-gooder; I'm just doing my best, and that's all you can do. I know there will be times when you will feel resentful, tearful, cross, frustrated and everything else in between, but every morning wake up and 'wipe the slate clean'. So please focus on the positive even if you're feeling really rotten. What I find helps is having something to look forward to – an outing, time with friends or a mini holiday.

Back in the 'good old days' when I didn't have any responsibility for anything other than myself and my cats, I could sleep in all morning and not even get dressed at the weekends. I didn't have to worry about having food in the fridge as I could order in a takeaway.

I didn't have 'strangers' (also known as carers) arriving on my doorstep at 8 or 9am and coming back again at 7pm – meaning that I had to at least be dressed. When the carers came in, this allowed me an hour to whizz around the supermarket to get food, toiletries and wine (for me!).

The carers look in your cupboards, the fridge when making meals and the airing cupboard. I often felt 'judged', even if they weren't judging me. There shouldn't be any 'out of date' food in the fridge, and oops I didn't do the ironing again. It felt like these 'strangers' they were my judge and jury!

It's so hard to accept help, but if you want to survive, you *need* these people. Your once quiet life where you had the freedom to do what you wanted, when you wanted, has now turned into a circus of routine, strangers and zero social life. But if you want the help from the carers, this comes at a cost.

Making time for you

This might sound selfish, but it's not; it's absolutely vital for your health and well-being. If you're not well and refreshed, there's no way you can help anybody else. During my times on duty 24/7 – more or less 365 days a year – I couldn't keep going with my health deteriorating and neither can you. Think of the safety checks given by a flight attendant when you're on a plane. Put the oxygen mask on yourself first, before helping others do the same.

Please don't be the person that arrives in their pink slippers to the GP. Take stock now before you become ill or exhausted.

CHAPTER 13

THE FEELING OF FREEDOM

May 2018

I'm sitting here in the sunshine with a light breeze, overlooking the Tramuntana mountains near Palma, Majorca. I feel a million light years away from home and my responsibilities.

The palm trees are gently moving, the air is so sweet, the birds are singing; I think I have found true paradise.

I've just spent a wonderful week with fabulous friends, strangers that I didn't know until last Saturday, in this beautiful part of the world, getting 'me' back. The 'old' Jane that used to be so full of joy, happy, as free as a bird; seeing friends and family, socialising and most of all laughing and enjoying all that life had to offer, or so I thought…

So, I'm sitting here in the middle of the Majorcan hills tapping away on my computer after spending one whole week getting *me* back. I'm not saying that the whole of me is back to where I want to be, but it's one heck of a start!

To be fair, after four years of caring for my Mum and 'trying' to live my life, plus work and all the family responsibilities that come with life, a week just isn't long enough. But I now have my mojo back and the skills and tools to support me on my journey – enjoying life once more.

I'm beginning to *feel* again. I'm not just a robot doing things for others, so much so that it didn't matter how I was doing!

In truth, prior to being here, I was not that bothered about me at all. I felt sad for what I had lost, not just Mum with her dementia, but *me*. I felt like my life had ended too with this awful disease, and at times I was past caring – I was just 'doing'.

I'm not saying I was depressed, but maybe I was; it seemed like each day it became harder and harder to get up in the morning and even harder to put on my 'happy face' and pretend that everything was OK.

When I mentioned the holiday to Claire, Mum's wonderful carer, she immediately said, '*Go*, I'll look after Mum. Go and have a fabulous time; you deserve a break.' In truth, Claire doesn't just look after Mum, but all of us. Claire admitted that she had been concerned about me for some time and had been trying in her own lovely way to tell me that I was burning out!

Freedom, space and time for me is what I was craving and that's why I have just loved this week away. I've let go of a lot of 'stuff', whether it be anxiety, depression, reliance on food, wine, diet coke, etc., but also had time just to think about nothing.

Gone are the 'To Do' lists. Routines, time and space have been given back to me in abundance. I had started to live life in a 'cell', or is that on a hamster wheel? The 'cell' is where I was locked into this life of routine, confinement and loneliness, and without a date for release. But also dreading that day.

As I head back and face reality once more, I feel I'm more equipped than ever to face the world head on. The break has done me the world of good. I'm busy planning my next break as we speak.

CHAPTER 14

MUM TODAY

Mum is almost 94 and living a contented life. She is not angry or sad any more. She loves her days and her normal routine.

As a reminder, almost four years ago she was falling all the time, doubly incontinent and had basically given up on life. Today she is not incontinent at all and she loves to go out and about, and enjoys it when friends come to see her, albeit just for a cup of tea and cake. Yes, she does get tired, but I think I will too if I reach her age. And yes she does get uppity when things don't always work as smoothly as they might, but don't we all on occasion?

It is clear that she has lost all memory from when she moved into her flat to when she came to live here (17 years), but she now remembers the old days and her short-term memory is a lot sharper than it used to be; especially if I have done something wrong, or if she did something nice over the last few days, which is lovely.

She remembers people's names and hasn't called me 'Mother' in three years. She is also far more aware of the day and time, but probably still couldn't tell you the year or the prime minister's name, but what does that matter?

But she does show an interest still in politics and looks forward to watching the news as she likes to know what's going on in the outside world; but she doesn't ponder or worry about things, as her world is warm, safe, secure and happy.

I'm blessed.

CONCLUSION

Thank you for taking the time to read *Pink Slippers*.

I hope my learnings and experience will be useful to any carer and their loved ones, to make their world a happier and healthier one. I am certainly no doctor nor do I have any medical/caring experience. This is just me – a normal everyday kind of person who has been thrown in at the deep end and is learning to live again.

I sincerely hope you've found some of the strategies, tips and comments helpful and I wish you every success with your loved one.

Please just remember that you are as important, if not more important, than your loved one – because without you, where would they be?

You are only human and you can only do as much as you can do. So please do not beat yourself up when times are hard; you are doing an extraordinary job and not just anyone can do what you are doing.

And please don't believe everything that others, including doctors, will tell you. Please question everything. The more you understand about the 'broken brain', the clearer things will be for you to make simple adjustments to help both you and your loved one.

Remember to take just one day at a time.

ABOUT ME – JANE HARDY

I was born in Bradford 57 years ago and adopted by a loving family at six weeks old. I was very blessed. It was no secret that I was adopted. In fact, I was made to feel like 'the chosen one', which made me feel very special indeed. My favourite memory of Mum and Dad was of them telling me how they chose me. They said that when they made the decision to adopt, they didn't know how they were going to choose. But they were taken into a large room where lots of babies lay in their cradles and when they saw me, they instantly knew I was the one because I was the prettiest baby there. What a wonderful story that was. Growing up I knew how much I was loved and wanted.

My parents Peter and Beth were told that they couldn't have children but nine months after adopting me, Mum fell pregnant with my sister Sarah. What a gift. I had an idyllic childhood; my first seven years we lived in Yorkshire near Harrogate and then we moved to Virginia Water in Surrey.

Growing up, I wasn't the brightest of children. After finishing my O levels, I decided to go to Brooklands Technical College to learn secretarial skills. Mum encouraged me and suggested that by having a skill I would always be able to earn a living, and she was right.

I really wanted to be a police motorcyclist, or so I thought. If the truth be known, I fancied Ian, a cadet policeman. Unfortunately, being 'vertically challenged' at 5'2", I was turned down by the police force when I was 16. I guess that wasn't the path for me. Nowadays though, I definitely see policemen and women shorter than me!

During my working career I started off as a secretary, worked my way up to an office manager and then went into marketing and customer services. By the time I was 30 I was in sales and managed my own team.

My last 'job' I had, I worked for a big American software company. I was the business development manager for Europe. This was my 'dream job', or so I thought. I loved my role and the team I managed. Life was good. I earned a fortune, travelled here, there and everywhere but one thing was missing – work/life balance.

What was the point of working so hard and not being able to enjoy the benefits? My life soon came crashing to a halt.

One morning I was due to give a presentation to an extremely large financial services organisation. I really wasn't feeling well. I was never ill. What was going on? I felt so bad that by the time I reached the hotel, I asked them to ring an ambulance for me. The ambulance crew arrived, took one look at me and said that I was having a panic attack – I told them in no uncertain terms that I didn't do panic attacks!

Rather to be safe than sorry, they decided to take me to Leeds General Infirmary (LGI). Talk about being in the right place at the right time. On the way to the hospital, I had a cardiac arrest. It turned out that I had arrhythmia; where my heart went into an abnormal rhythm.

I didn't see that coming! I spent two weeks in the LGI and was fitted with an implantable cardioverter defibrillator (a posh pacemaker!). My ICD is affectionately called Doris – my angel on my shoulder. Doris's job is to keep me alive. Should my heart ever decide to go into a crazy rhythm again, Doris will give me a little shock to get my heart back into a normal rhythm.

Today, I'm on Doris number three. I also have Horace! Horace is the clever computer at home that 'talks' to Doris. He sends all the data from Doris wirelessly to St George's in Tooting so that they can keep an eye on me! Nothing like 'Big Brother' watching you!

I feel so humbled and blessed to be in the care of the NHS. I have nothing but praise for the NHS, particularly St George's and the staff there. Such incredible human beings doing an incredible job. People moan about the NHS but I can't fault them.

I do believe that in life we are often presented with challenges that force us to change our path. After my recovery, I lost all my confidence, was petrified of my own shadow. I became agoraphobic.

Everything changed in an instant.

One minute I was flying around Europe without a care in the world, delivering presentations, sealing deals for the company. The next minute I was too scared to leave my home. I was scared stiff. What if 'Doris' went off, or worse still, what if 'Doris' didn't go off and I dropped down dead?

My illness became so bad that I ended up being admitted to The Priory with post-traumatic stress disorder. Thank goodness for the medical insurance that covered the cost of my stay.

Soon after my ordeal, it was pretty clear that I was no longer a 'someone' at work. In big corporate firms, you become a name and number and if you no longer perform to their standards, you are basically 'thrown out to the wolves'. That was a very painful time in my life.

When dealing with a life-changing condition, you begin to question yourself over and over again, and why me? When I had that cardiac arrest 14 years ago, there was only a 5% survival rate. So why had I survived? All I kept thinking was that I wasn't ready to die yet; I still had so much to give. I had to find my purpose.

This is where I discovered business networking – where many small business owners come together to share their ideas and help each other to grow their own business. As I mentioned earlier, Fabulous Networking is one of those such organisations – www.fabulousnetworking.co.uk. I owned this company for five years and grew it to 30 groups across the South East, but just before Christmas 2018, as it was growing so quickly I decided to sell it to give more time for me and Mum.

I am now an entrepreneur involved with various smaller projects and of course writing and spending more time with my family.

And one of the best things of all is actually having time for me too and I have just joined a rock singing group (www.singingrockclub.co.uk), which I love and gives me a feeling of freedom and fun.

USEFUL WEBSITES AND RESOURCES

Facebook: Dementia Carers Support Group UK: www.facebook.com/groups/1935237626700874

There are many support groups on Facebook, but I love this one. You can shout, cry and ask for help and you will get so much support from your peers.

Facebook: Fabulous Carers: This is a closed carers' support group for those who have read my book and are asking for help and advice. www.facebook. com/groups/FabulousCarers

Age UK: www.ageuk.org.uk

My favourite website which gives help and advice on dementia and where to get support.

Alzheimer's Society: www.alzheimers.org.uk

Full of useful information and contacts for help.

Crossroads: www.crossroadscaresurrey.org.uk

Crossroads helps support both the carer and loved one – from respite care and clubs to end-of-life support.

Gumtree: www.gumtree.com

A website where you could potentially find carers, without going through a Care Agency.

Please claim Attendance Allowance if your loved one has dementia – www.gov.uk/attendance-allowance. This website will also give you advice on other benefits.

A recommended book is: *The 36-Hour Day – A Family Guide to Caring for People Who Have Alzheimer Disease, Other Dementias and Memory Loss* – by Nancy L Mace and Peter V Rabins.

An easy-to-read and clear description of dementia by the NHS: www.nhs.uk/conditions/dementia/about

A helpline and support from Admiral Nurses: www.dementiauk.org/get-support